Survival Guide:
20 Strategies To Survive In The Wilderness During The Cold Season

Table of content

Introduction

Our daily lives are super dependent on technology and readily available food at all times. We have fine homes with heaters and gas stoves to serve us with ease and comfort. What if one day all of it was taken away from you and you were to survive, out in the wilderness and that too in extreme winter season? Sounds adventurous right? It is easier said than done. Surviving out there in the wild isn't the easiest of things to do. Not just your comfort and health is at risk, it's a matter of survival or giving up to simply die.

The survival skills become highly essential. Yes, they do come naturally in times of intense need but they should be known, understood, well-practiced and well-executed. Out there in the wild, you face all kinds of odds. You're faced with extreme harsh, skin biting cold trying to get in you and freeze you. One the other hand, you are as vulnerable as anything is in the wild. There would be animals of your size or may be even bigger than you. Would you simply let all these factors take you down and surrender? The answer should be a definite no.

A human is made far smarter than anything around us. Our natural survival instincts take us farther than anybody has ever gone. Knowing the strategies and the skills required to execute these strategies will play a vital role in your survival out there in the wilderness. Watched Leo's The Revenant? You might need to go to pretty much the same extent in extreme cases.

Either you're out on an adventure or are stuck in the wilderness, make sure you have the right tools with you to make your survival possible. The wilderness can offer odds beyond human control, thus, knowing and applying the methods to make your survival extended would be critical.

Chapter 1 – Basics of Survival in the Wilderness in Winter

Winter is the season where all the travelers make a plan for the activities such as climbing, hiking, camping outdoor and much more. It is the season where preparation and planning are at the peak of those people who love to stay outdoor. It is not easy to survive in the wilderness during the winter seasons which is why you need to know the basics of it which are essential. You need to have the proper information so that you do not end up getting in trouble since everything would be roaming around outside.

You need to have certain clothes which will keep you warm and alertness so no animal can attack you. You need to have sharp hearing practice, so you can judge if something is approaching your anything dangerous is on your way. It is a risk if you are going to the wilderness on your own the first time. When you get experienced, then it turns out to be a trip full of fun. The best thing is to go with lots of people so you can enjoy and everyone supports each other.

You need to know some of the basics to get started with the wilderness which are as followings:

1. *Shelter*

You need to build a shelter such as a camp where you can stay during the night time. You have to sleep obviously so make sure you are covered properly from all the surroundings, and you can sleep safe and sound. Pick an area which is away from the crowd of wilderness and calm. You can also find a cave and stay there, but that will be happening when you are too acquainted with the place. There should be enough airflow for you to survive in the wilderness.

2. Set Fire

To keep yourself warm, you will have to set the fire in the woods. That will be the fun part where you will learn how to set fire in the woods by yourself. You can survive through the fireplace being near you during the winters for sure. You have to keep your body warm despite wearing warm clothes or drinking the warm stuff. The fireplace can be a big rescue for you in the winters. You have to make a pit and then put the wood logs in it. Make sure you stay away while doing all this because fire can be dangerous.

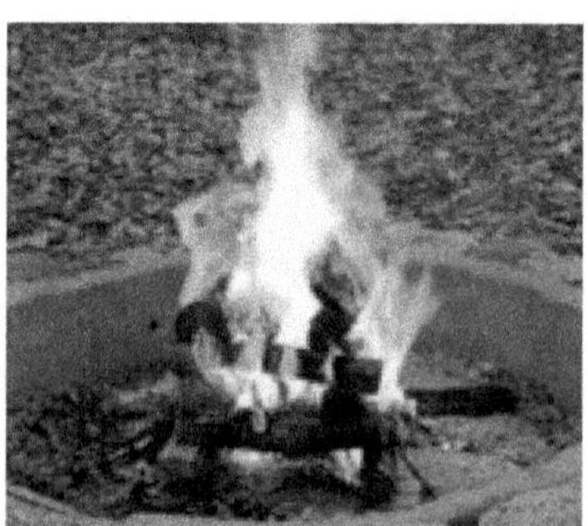

3. First Aid

You need to have the first aid kit with you and the basics through which you can support your friend or family when they are feeling sick. Sometimes, the cold weather can effect so bad that the condition can get severe of the person such as breathing or flu, fever and much more. You need to keep the necessary things in the first aid kit and know how to use them. You should be aware of knowing how to handle a situation by keeping everything under consideration so that in your presence you can take care of the person fully and responsibly.

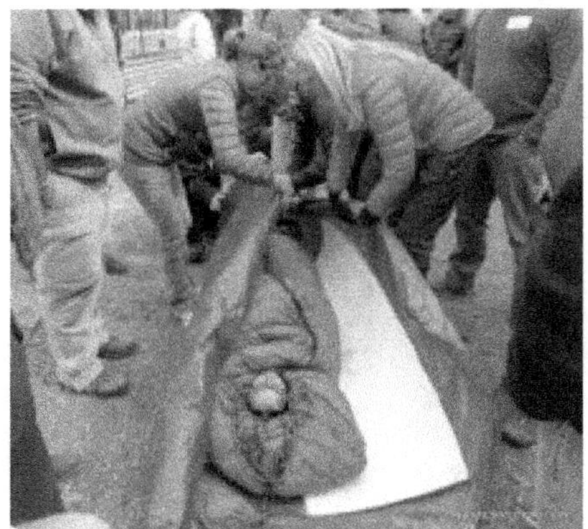

4. Keep it moisture around you

Make sure to melt the snow which is around you because if it is frozen, then you will feel colder. So make sure to keep the snow melted by the fire or reside at a place where there is not much of the pile of snow. You can put the snow into a bottle and then melt it by keeping it warm under your coat so it can melt. You can also keep it near the fire and make pure water out of it to drink it. So basically you will not be hydrated if you try the option for melting snow. You cannot survive without water so make sure to keep abundance of it. You may be able to survive without food for some days but without water, the survival will be hard.

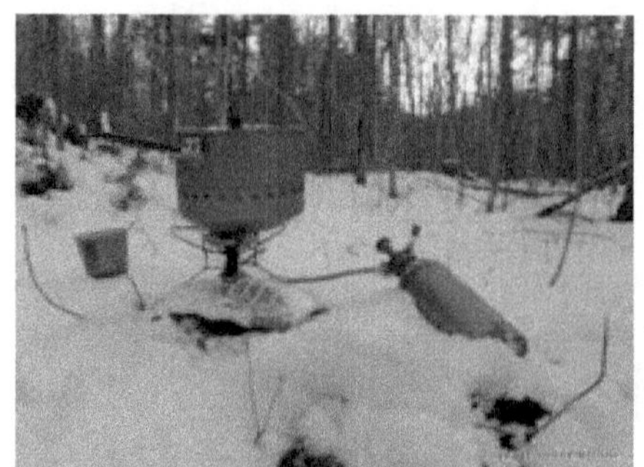

Chapter 2 – Strategies to Build Fire and Shelter in Winter

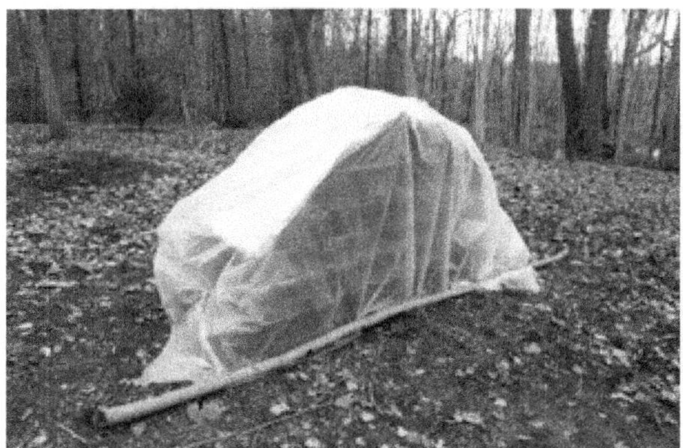

There are different types of shelter which you can make when you are trying to survive in the winter wilderness. It is easy, but since you are there for long, then you need to make sure to make a strong one which can sustain for longer days and you do not have to put it back again after a while. If you are giving time to it, then make sure to build a proper shelter which can provide you all the ease and comfort while staying outdoor.

Here are some of the ways which you can build the shelter easily. Shelters need to be safe so that you can sleep in it properly. Most of the people get confused that when you are sleeping outdoor, you cannot have a deep sleep due to the fear that something might attack you at night, but that is not the case. You can set some signs which can guide you when something is approaching you so that you wake up and be alert at the same time.

5. Make Frame

You have to build the frame first to get started with it. If the frame is strong, then all the shelter will stay for many days. Even if cold winds hit your shelter, it won't come off. You will be warm in your shelter. You have to secure the sides and the corners by making it wider.

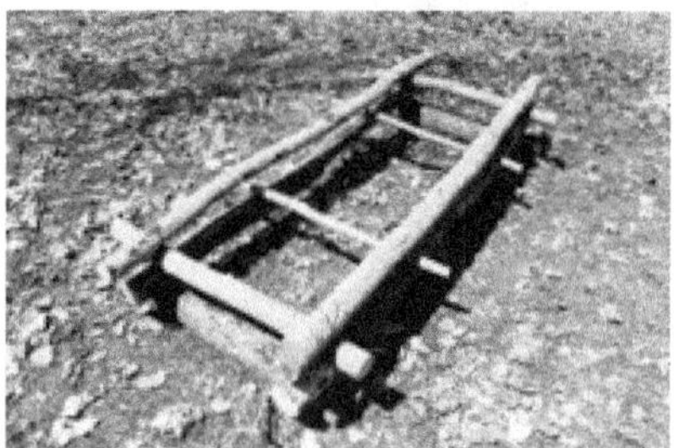

6. Make the bottom – bed

You have to make a pattern whichever you like to make the bottom of the bed. There are many styles of bedding which you can make whichever is comfortable for you. Make the firm bottom so that you do not have to sleep directly on the ground.

7. *Make the Framework*

Now you have to make the roof of the shelter now so you can choose if you want it straight or you want it round. The round will be better because it will keep it warm and cozy. Make sure to keep it cozy so that you are comfortable staying inside. Here is an example how you can make the roof of the shelter.

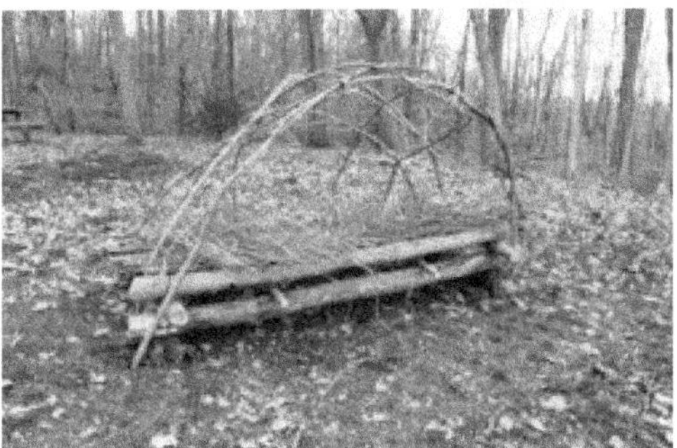

8. *Cover the Shelter*

The last part is to cover the shelter by binding it from all the sides. You have to make sure you tie the knots completely so that it cannot come off. Make sure to keep it secure with the thick cloth so that you are warm inside. Even if you wear warm clothes, then you still need to stay at the place which is comfortable. To make the shelter, you need to have proper supplies to get it done completely. So do it carefully and step by step and you will realize how awesome the shelter will be.

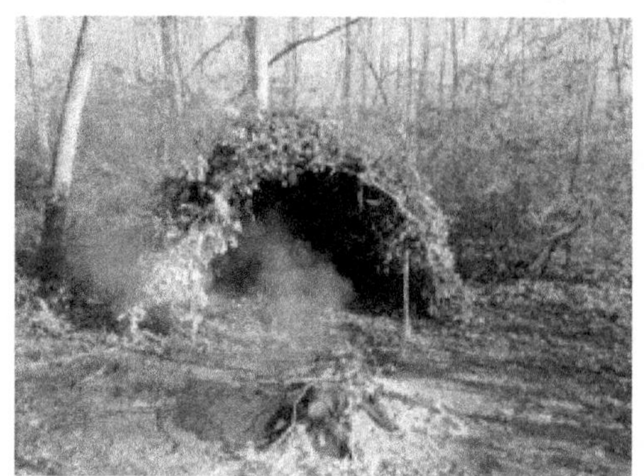

Chapter 3 – Strategies to Set Traps and Get Food

When you are in the wilderness, it is obvious that you cannot get the proper food which you get from the stores like your home. You need to know how to set the traps for the animals and cook food out of them. It can be hard, but the adventure is never easy. You need to get out of your comfort zone to learn more about it. You will be feeling hungry more than usual since it is winter and in winters, you have to stay warm, so you need to eat. The easiest way to get the food is to access the wild plants. There are many vegetables which you can have and make them over the fire in a pot. You can also gather animals and cook meat. You can hunt and make food for yourself by trapping the right animals which you can eat.

9. *How to find the food*

Eating is a matter in which no one can compromise. You have to make sure that the meat which you catch, you can swallow it and it would suit your body. You have to take off the skin of the animals by yourself which are edible. You have to cook the meat which gives you enough protein and keep you energized. Make sure to get the right weapons which you can hunt from.

Almost any healthy human being can very well get along without food for a few days and would only feel hunger and some stomach cramps as a result of it. Mostly in winters, the edible vegetables are not so easily available to be consumed, so we'll discuss becoming a smart hunter to gather animal food here. Animal meat in the wild would fulfill the hunger needs and satisfy body requirements of food to survive in the wilderness. Let's dive into some interesting techniques on hunting and setting traps.

10.Survival Food Search:

Your dietary preferences should be the least of your concern when eating becomes a matter of life and death, especially if you're stranded in the wilderness for an extended period. Virtually, all mammals are edible except for a few who can't be used as safe food. However, it is essential to know that eating creatures which appear weak should be avoided. Cooking the meat is highly advised if possible. Also, high protein sources such as cicadas, katydids, crickets and grasshoppers shouldn't be left alone.

11. Use of Primitive Weapons:

You can use a sturdy hunk of the branch and can use it as a very basic throwing stick to strike an animal. IT could ideally be half the thickness of your wrist and approximately about 2 and a half feet long. It should be broken in this size for it to be effective as a weapon.

You can use it to throw at a further range like an arrow or strike it sideways to bring down a squirrel on the side of a tree. In the first method, your left foot should be pointing towards the target. It could be vice versa in case you're a left handed person. Afterward, hold the smaller end of the stick loosely, stretching the weapon back of your shoulder and throw it spinning towards the target.

Make sure you're always carrying a well-sharpened throwing stick when you're camping for any good reason. Not only you'll have a chance to bring down an animal or a bird, but you can also knock down nuts or fruit from trees with the same club.

Any abrupt movements should be avoided to talk well. Walk fairly slow and make sure your feet feel the ground. Coincide your movements with the feeding pattern of animals around you. Most of the animals, while collecting food, look around and scan for any potential dangers they might encounter. However, this is easier said than done. You require practice to get an expert level command in using the club to intend your survival streak.

12. *The Snare Trap:*

Using primarily foraged materials in the wilderness setting, there are probably well over 100 traps that can be fashioned with it. Although, every student of outdoor survival would be well acquainted or advised about knowing as many as they possibly can. However, the most famous, easily made and versatile ones are Figure 4 Deadfall and the rolling snare.

A snare is positioned in such a manner that it can lasso and animal, mostly killing it instantly by breaking their neck. It's a little more than a nose, made up of string, handwoven cordage or sinew. It could be placed at a well-known animal trail. Make sure that you put it in an appropriate place because if an animal bigger than anticipated gets tangled, it will most likely destroy the trap.

13. *Deadfall Trap:*

When triggered, a deadfall/baited trap drops weight on the animal and killing it right away. The figure 4 trap is as simple as many other traps. It has three sticks.

When the trap is used for rabbit sized animals, two of these sticks should be about six inches long. The third one should be nearing 8 inches. The sizes could be adjusted depending on the animal on the catching list. The weight is usually a big log or a flattish rock.

Never directly in a run or line of travel. Remember when assembling it that the vertical stake should not be positioned beneath the rock or log, that the bait should be attached to the crosspiece and as far under the weight as is practical, and that a small fence of twigs around the outer portion of the upright can prevent an animal from inadvertently setting off the device by striking the trigger while not under the log or rock.

14. Trapping:

You should focus on selecting areas with high game activity including sources of water and where the forest meets meadow and fields. In these areas, you're very likely to spot specific runs, feeding areas, lays, day beds, and trails. Once you've identified the spot, you can place your trap for the best results. However, when you're out in the wild, you'll for sure face some exceptions which are beyond human rules.

The traps will help you catch the right for you which you can cook and have dinner with your friends and family. You do not have to eat vegetables all the time, but you can also hunt the animals and serve yourself some good dinner. You just need to have the right equipment and tools which can help you in hunting the animals. Sometimes when you are inexperienced, you tend to hunt it, but that animal is still alive which can be dangerous for you. So you need to make sure you know how to hunt before you go ahead with living in the wilderness. It requires a lot of research and practice when you plan to survive in the wilderness. So if you are a newbie then do not go alone but along with a lot of people so that you have some support for yourself.

Chapter 4 – Strategies to Keep Your Body Warm in Winter

Staying comfortable and warm while Hiking, snow shoeing, backcountry skiing or Nordic is a significant challenge. Yes, we do sweat, but it makes our clothes damp, increasing the chances of catching a cold. However, staying warm in such harsh conditions isn't impossible. There are some brilliant tricks that are tried and tested over the years by experts who are winter freaks but also are smart in their brain. These tips will make getting outdoor in winter way more easy, enjoyable and comfortable for everyone of you. Follow these tips to make the most of your winter outdoor trips and enjoy to the fullest in your adventures.

15. Move Around:

Clothing traps only your body heat. Ultimately, it's your body temperature that regulates to keep you warm and cozy. While you're outdoor and you're beginning to feel cold, the best method to shake it off is to start moving or move faster and increase your pace. Look out for signs of your team members, family or friends that they are feeling cold, especially children, who have to get colder faster because of less body fat and mass as compared to adults. When you take a break, make sure its short to avoid cooling down your body temperature.

16. Set Your Pace

To stay warm, it is critical to minimizing the level of perspiring in cold temperatures as the heat from your body is conducted away from wet clothes. Adjust your pace in such a way that helps you stay warm without overheating and heavily perspiring. If you don't want to go to slow and sweating in unavoidable, as you get closer to the top, reduce your pace to a level where your sweating stops but still enough heat is produced to dry out your base layers. It can be done 20 to 30 minutes before stopping to camp.

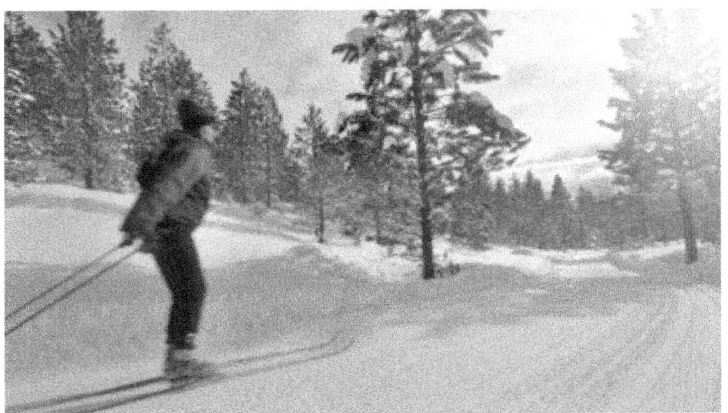

17. Layers Adjustment

Avoid sweat in high-exertion activities like Nordin skiing or running becomes inevitable. As a result, you need to adjust the layers of your clothing. If for example, there's no wind and you're putting in some real exertion, you may only require an insulation layer which is breathable, over a wicking and fast-drying base layer. If in case, it is windy, you might need to take on a breathable waterproof hard shell on top of a midweight layer of insulation, like a vest or fleece to prevent yourself from bringing your body temperature down.

18.Eat More:

In freezing temperatures, the body needs more fuel to keep your internal furnace heated up and burning. High-fat snacks like nuts and chocolate are recommended since fat burns slowly and keep your body going for a longer stride, which gets even more important as survival in the cold.

19.Drink Up

In colder temperatures, our body gets dehydrated more quickly than we realize even if you're not sweating too much. Keep a hot drink in a thermos and drink frequently. Add a little dollop of butter for fat and flavor or add a bit of sugar for instant energy.

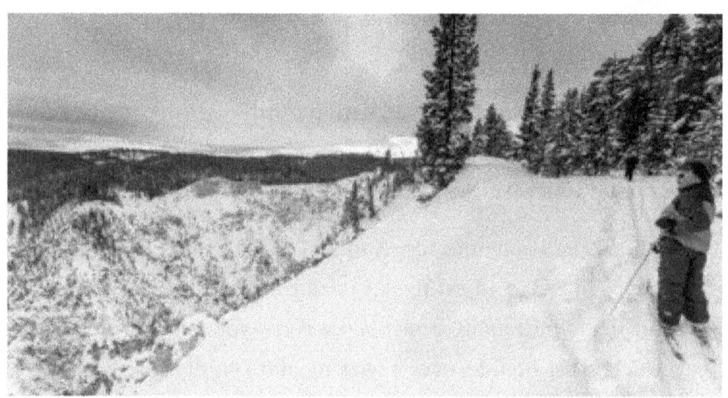

20.Don't Freeze Your Water

Make sure your water doesn't freeze. Keep it under your hood and upside down. In case there's any ice accumulated, it will be at the bottom instead of the top. In further freezing temperatures, make sure you don't leave your water supplies outside since they will freeze within no time. Either empty your bottles, or also, you can fill them with hot water and use inside as heaters in your sleeping bag.

Keep Spare Gloves

Do your fingers get easily cold and are difficult to warm again? The solution is to carry an extra pair of gloves and keep the spare in your jacket pocket near the torso so that they remain warm and toasty. Once your hands get cold and frozen, remove the pair of gloves you're wearing and warm your hands in your pant pockets or against your belly. Wear the extra gloves and put these cold ones back in your jacket pocket so that the cycle continues as long as you're out in the wilderness.

Mittens are, however, warmer than gloves as their collective warmth keeps the fingers warm and cozy. Whenever in extreme cold, mittens are highly preferred to be worn instead of gloves or you can wear them on top of your light gloves.

Keep Two Hats:

It's a good idea to keep two hats. One could be a really warm hat and a slightly lighter one. You can use the warm one while you're snowshoeing downhill, skiing or resting. Similarly, while you're in moderately cold temperatures and don't want a super warm hat, use the lighter one that you carried so that you don't get overheated.

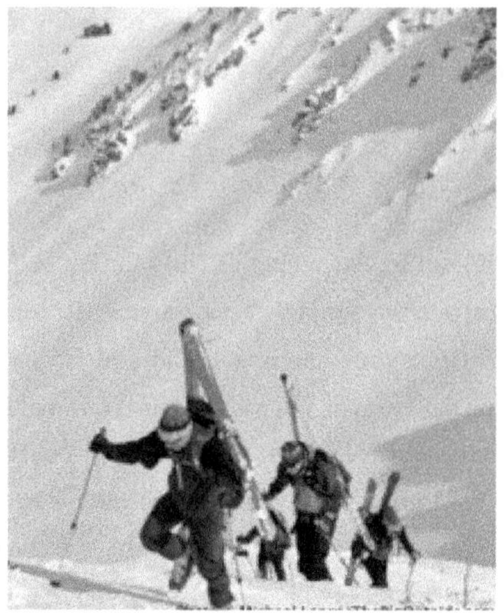

Sit On Your Pack

The logs, rocks, ground and all other objects are frozen in winter, and when you make contact with them, they will suck the heat from your body. It's called thermal conduction. As an alternate, you can put your pack down on the cold ground and use it for sitting.

When your body is warm, you feel better which is why it is really important for you to survive in the winters. Think about your safety before anything else. Our bodies feel cold when we are not eating well, or we do not keep it warm. So when you are moving for an outdoor trip, keep all kind of warm clothes which can help you stay warm and you can enjoy fully. When you keep yourself warm, you will be away from catching any diseases such as flu or fever which is common when people feel cold. Do not ruin your trip by getting sick so make sure to get the right things packed which can keep you safe and warm in the cold winter nights.

You need to keep the night suit which is warm as well because when the sun sets, the night gets colder. So do not wait and start collecting the jackets, gloves and especially the boots, so you can walk with warm feet. If your feet is warm, then your whole body temperature stays normal.

Chapter 5 – Strategies to Find Way in the Wilderness in Winter Season

Everything seems to be in order in the best case scenario; charged iPhone with all the apps in the world. However, the things don't seem so easy and refined when you're injured, or your phone's battery is dead. There are a few skills you need to learn which are inevitable in helping you out when your dependence on the digital items has failed you. These tips will make you realize that people survived in the past too, without these digital helpers alongside. Creek Stewart, a survival expert, has tested himself with real life scenarios and situations where he survived as a part of his training and wishes others to be similarly competent and strong enough to make sure that the survival instincts are up and running in case of need.

There are countless books and videos on YouTube which you can read or watch all day long but the hands-on experience that one gets while getting out in the wilderness and letting the natural will survive take over, a person learns way more as compared to the artificial environment. This book will provide Stewart's proven skills which will raise your ultimate limits of survival techniques.

You can now practice and master these amazing tactics to stay safe in the wilderness. Take a friend who loves outdoors and get on for some brilliant Blackwood experience. Make sure you let your friends and family know about your exact whereabouts before taking off!

Look out for a suitable campsite:

Your goal should be to stay dry and high as guided by Stewart as well. Avoid pathways and valleys where there's a high chance that water may travel towards you. That's why flash-floods are famous for covering a low-lying area in a matter of minutes. Select a campsite which is free from dangers such as insect nests, dead branches which can come down any time as well as rocks traveling down due to land sliding. Preferably, the best place to set your camp is near dry wood which can be used for shelter and fire both. Also, your camp should be near the running water.

Build a Shelter:

The number one killer in cold weather is what we call hypothermia. This means that in a prolonged survival situation, your top priority should be a well-insulated shelter. Look out for a tree which is downed at an angle or set branches across a standing tree along with smaller branches closely on the opposite side. Set upon a good layer of debris on the floor which is most likely to suck all your heat. The debris could be comprised of leaves or moss, nearly 4 to 5 inches to block any cold reaching up to you while you're lying. Also, make sure the angled wall is set across with debris as well.

Starting a fire using battery:

Any battery will do just fine since we have to short-circuit the battery. Take a wire and connect with it the positive and negative terminals, wrapped in a gum wrapper and this should have your firewood ready.

Keeping the Fire Burning:

There are primarily four ingredients which will help you to keep your fire growing and burning. Firstly, fibrous material of dried tinder bundle, for example, a cotton balls which are covered in lip balm or Vaseline are a brilliant choice in case you have them and three sized wood; pencil, q-tip, and toothpick. Use a wood log of a forearm size to be used as a windscreen and base for your tender. As soon as the tinder is lit, stack the smaller log against the larger log in a leaning position so that the oxygen passes through the flames. Add Kindles which are larger until the fire grows hot enough for bigger wood logs.

Finding Clean Drinking Water:

In the wild, you'll come across two kinds of water. One which is potable water can be used for drinking as it's already purified. However, the other kind can simply kill you. Questionable water could be anything that's stagnant for a long term like a puddle or streams. The best option is to boil which may not be an option to carry out in the wild!

Dew, rain, and snow are pure and reliable sources of water which can be used for drinking. Surprisingly, it can be collected with a lot of ease too. They are already purified. You can use a couple of your bandanas to take snow in it and squeeze them to collect a significant amount of clean drinkable water. If there are any maple trees around, Cut a hole in its bark, and you'll have one the best watery syrup energy drink available, straight from nature.

Conclusion

Surviving in the wilderness can be hard which is why you need to be very careful and find out the proper steps. After reading this eBook, you must be able to build the shelter and set the traps to have proper food for your survival. You cannot survive without food for more than three days which is why even if you take enough food with you, you will still have to find the food in the wilderness and cook it yourself. You need to make sure to get the food which is clean and eatable. Do not hunt the animals which you think you cannot consume.

Being careful in the wilderness is the main thing. You are new to the environment, so you have to be alert all the time. Make sure to plan the trip with your friends and family so that you have the support of each other. You can share information with them, and they can also share their knowledge about it. By having this eBook with you all the time, you will be able to plan properly and accordingly without getting confused. You will understand where you need to take which steps so that you do not miss out on any things.

When you are not aware of anything, then it gets tough to survive which is why you need to make sure that you read it carefully and if you want to memorize it then note down some of the important points which you think you will need. You do not have to go through a hard time or not figure out what is happening so do not hesitate to learn from this eBook. It will work as a great favor for you to get started or even plan to live well in the wilderness during the winter season.

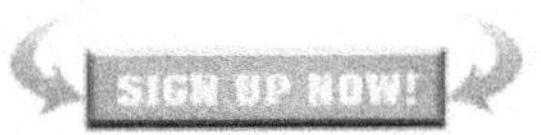

OR Go to this URL

http://zbit.ly/1WBb1Ek

www.ingramcontent.com/pod-product-compliance
Lightning Source LLC
Chambersburg PA
CBHW061928270726
48660CB00003BA/1104